Write for Wellness
Write Your Way to Health, Healing and Happiness

Elaine Beale

ISBN: 9781797405964

CONTENTS

INTRODUCTION

"Writing is medicine. It is an appropriate antidote to injury. It is an appropriate companion for any difficult change."
Julia Cameron, *The Artist's Way.*

Who Is This Book For?

Have you ever found yourself wondering why you don't do what you *know* is good for your health? Regular exercise, for example? Or eating less sugar? Or getting enough sleep?

Or perhaps you suffer with anxiety and have yet to find a way to manage it. Or maybe you had a traumatic experience that continues to upset you or weigh on your mind.

Perhaps you have a chronic illness or condition that impacts your daily living. Or perhaps you are the caretaker of an ill or aging family member and find yourself feeling isolated or overwhelmed. Or maybe you are struggling to come to terms with a death or the loss of something of great importance to you, like a marriage or a job.

Or perhaps you simply want to improve your relationships and live a fuller, more joyous and satisfying life.

If any of these things are true for you, writing can help you. It can help you understand what gets in the way of committing to your own wellness and help you to make positive changes. It can reduce your anxiety and worry. It can help you resolve traumatic or difficult past experiences. It can also improve your sleep, relieve symptoms of chronic illness, and help you come to terms with grief and loss. It can provide you with insights about your life and the meaning and significance of your past experiences. And it can help you change your mindset and outlook so you can be more optimistic and less likely to engage in negative self-talk.

What's the Evidence?

Understandably, you may be a little skeptical about these claims, but they are all founded on scientific evidence. In fact, there have been numerous studies that have looked at the impact of what is known as expressive writing[1] on many aspects of health and wellness. And, as I detail in Chapter One of this book, these studies have demonstrated that writing is a powerful tool that can improve your health and well-being. In fact, if writing were a pill, you can bet that all the pharmaceutical companies would be advertising it heavily and selling it to millions of satisfied customers throughout the world.

Instead, unlike most medications, writing is free. And, unlike the drugs we see advertised on television, there's no long list of scary side-effects. What's more, as long as you have pen and paper (or a computer or tablet), you can do it. What's more, once you learn the techniques outlined in this book, you can use it wherever and whenever you want.

I know about writing's positive effects on health, mood and mindset because I have used it myself. I also know about it because for more than 25 years I have taught writing as a tool to support wellness and healing at community organizations, educational institutions, and private workshops.

My own writing practice helped me heal from a traumatic childhood, deal with depression, and develop tools to manage a chronic illness. I also relied on writing to help me get through the sudden death of my mother and the slow decline of my father from Alzheimer's Disease. For me, writing has been a kind of salvation. It may not have literally saved my life, but it has certainly allowed me to live one that is healthier, more satisfying and happier.

How I Developed the Program

It was because I understood the transformational power of writing early in my writing career that I co-founded *Fearless Words*, a program designed to help survivors of sexual assault heal through writing. The program was sponsored by San Francisco Women Against Rape and received funding from the San Francisco Arts Commission for several years.

Before establishing *Fearless Words*, I anticipated that it would offer great benefits to participants, but I was truly amazed by the shifts that happened each time we offered the eight-week program. In the process of writing about trauma, long-held secrets, shame, anger, and other difficult emotions, participants took enormous steps towards healing. Writing allowed them to discharge negative feelings and created the possibility for a new understanding of their experiences. They let go of shame because they came to understand that they had no reason to feel shame for being assaulted. Self-blame was replaced by self-compassion. Some participants

---

[1] Expressive writing is a form of writing that is personal. It expresses emotions and describes experiences without regard to what form it is written in and without regard to writing conventions like spelling, grammar, and punctuation. In discussing writing throughout this book, I am referring to expressive writing.

stopped letting their anger eat away at them and chose instead to channel it into activism or community service. For many, the burden of carrying a secret was released and they felt a new sense of calm.

Of course, part of the transformation that occurred during *Fearless Words* was because of the connections participants made with each other and the way their experiences were normalized by sharing them with other survivors. However, I had run talk-based support groups for survivors of trauma prior to establishing *Fearless Words*, and those groups did not appear to result in the more profound healing that I saw result from writing.[2]

After seeing the remarkable results experienced by participants in *Fearless Words*, I went on to run other groups and workshops that used writing as a tool for wellness and healing. I've worked with people with chronic illness and disabilities, people who are grieving, LGBT people dealing with the negative impacts of social stigma and oppression, and people who simply want to develop greater self-awareness and improve the quality of their lives. In all cases, I've seen people transformed by the power of writing.

Later, I went on to create *Write Well!*, a program that combines evidence-based approaches using expressive writing for wellness with the methods I developed through my workshops. I decided to write this book because I wanted to make the *Write Well!* methods accessible and useable to a greater number of people.

I'm Not a Writer—Can This Book Help Me?

To benefit from this book, you do not have to consider yourself a writer. The majority of people I've worked with were not interested in writing for publication. When they began working with me, many expressed a lack of comfort with writing. Some were wary of writing because they'd had bad experiences at school that made them doubt their ability to express themselves through written language. Others were worried because they were not completely comfortable with the rules of grammar or spelling. Some thought that they didn't have the talent they assumed was required to write. Some had learning disabilities like dyslexia and felt self-conscious about putting words on the page. None of this mattered.

What did matter was that they were willing to approach the exercises in the way I instructed, and, as much as possible, to put aside their own critical voices or concern about what someone else might think about what they wrote. I recognize that this is not always easy. But it becomes easier

---

[2] Writing as part of a group of supportive individuals has great benefits, but as I describe later, you don't need to write in a group to experience the positive results of writing, and there is enough guidance in this book for you to complete the exercises alone. However, in Chapter Ten, I provide detailed guidance for anyone who may be interested in establishing a wellness, health or healing writing group.

with practice. And it's important to remember that the writing you will do when you use this book is not for anyone else. It is for you.

If you do decide to share what you write with someone else, that's fine. This book includes instructions about how to form a wellness writing group if that's an interest of yours. But whether you write alone or in a group with others is your decision. And, as I'll discuss in Chapter Two, it's important that, when you are engaged in writing, that you don't try to censor yourself or worry about an audience or reader.

There are many reasons why I encourage people to use the exercises in this book. First of all, the evidence strongly suggests that writing supports wellness, healing and health. You don't even have to devote a lot of time to it—most of the exercises in this book are short. And, as I describe in Chapter One, several studies have shown that just four 15-minute writing sessions can have a measurable impact on people's health!

What's more, you can do it when you want and almost anywhere—on the bus, in bed, during your lunch hour or coffee break. And while many people with disabilities, debilitating illnesses or caregiving responsibilities may find it difficult to attend a support group or be unable to afford therapy, most will find writing an easy way to support their health.

How to Use This Book
To make this book accessible, I've made it relatively short and easy to follow. In Chapter One, I discuss the evidence showing that writing is effective in improving health, wellness and positive mindset. I also talk about what we know so far about how and why it works. In Chapter Two, I talk about the methods you need to use to get the most out of the exercises in the rest of the book.

Chapter Three provides a wide variety of writing techniques and exercises to support overall wellness. Chapters Four through Eight provide exercises and writing methods to address specific areas of health and wellness, including living with chronic illness and pain, dealing with grief and loss, healing from trauma, developing a positive outlook, and creating healthy relationships at home and work. Chapter Nine includes several exercises anyone can use for personal development and self-insight. Chapter Ten provides guidelines to anyone interested in forming an expressive writing group to support wellness or a specific aspect of health.

You do not have to read this book from start to finish. For example, you may not be interested in the studies that I discuss in Chapter One, and you may feel that the chapter on dealing with grief and loss does not apply to you. Feel free to skip those chapters. <u>But make sure to read Chapter Two so you know how to approach the exercises.</u>

I hope you find this book a helpful guide and that, like me and so many of the people I've had the honor to work with, you come to appreciate the power of writing to help you create lasting improvements in your health and your life.

Elaine Beale

CHAPTER ONE
THE COMPELLING CASE FOR WRITING AS A TOOL FOR WELLNESS

"The scientific research on the benefits of so-called expressive writing is surprisingly vast. Studies have shown that writing about oneself and personal experiences can improve mood disorders, help reduce symptoms among cancer patients, improve a person's health after a heart attack, reduce doctor visits and even boost memory."

New York Times, January 19, 2015

The Power of Words

People have known for centuries that writing is a powerful tool that supports wellness, improves health, and promotes healing. By confiding their deepest feelings and hardest secrets to the page, people across the centuries and from all walks of life have been able to live fuller and happier lives.

For some who've experienced terrible trauma, loss, or isolation, writing made the difference between life and death. Just google the phrase, "Writing saved my life," and you'll find literally thousands of instances of people talking about how they were able to survive extremely challenging experiences through the act of writing. Some of those people are well known writers, but most are individuals who wrote only for themselves in private journals.

Those of us who are readers are also familiar with the power of the written word. Many of us have had the experience of reading a memoir or a work of fiction and suddenly feeling that the writer is capturing our own emotions and providing new and important insights into our lives. What you may not realize if you are not a writer is that authors themselves frequently gain new insights through the process of writing. Even when writing about major events in their own lives, the author may not have understood their significance prior to writing about them; the insights were only revealed to them through the act of writing itself.

As I'll discuss in more detail later in this chapter, it's only as we go about putting things into language that we are able to interpret our experience and give it greater meaning. Far more than talking, using written language to describe and understand events, problems or emotions opens a channel to our deepest selves. It allows us insight, greatly increases our capacity for problem solving, and allows us to reshape our own life narrative to allow more self-compassion, and give us a greater sense of purpose.

It may seem surprising that the psychological changes that result from writing can also have significant effects on our physical health. After all, western medicine has generally viewed the mind and body as separate entities and, as a result, we've been encouraged to see our mental and physical health are two entirely different things. But in the wake of new discoveries in neuroscience, this separation is being questioned. It turns out that what happens in the mind has an immense impact on the body, and what happens in the body has an immense impact on the mind.

So, if writing can allow people to make emotional and psychological shifts, it makes sense that it might also affect our physical well-being. Fortunately, we no longer have to speculate about this because numerous researchers have taken a look at the evidence. What they discovered is compelling.

The Evidence

It was during the late 1980s that social scientists, medical researchers and others began investigating whether the healing power of writing could actually be measured. Two of the first and most well-known researchers in this area are James Pennebaker and Joshua Smyth. In their book, *Opening Up by Writing It Down*, Pennebaker and Smyth discuss the earliest studies in which college students were asked to write for 15 minutes a day over four consecutive days. One group of students was asked to write about "the most upsetting or traumatic experience of your life" while a control group was asked to write about superficial topics, such as describing their dorm room in detail.

What struck the researchers first was that the students who had been asked to write about a trauma wrote about profound and often disturbing life events. These included parental divorce, sexual abuse, suicide attempts, and family alcoholism. For this group, following the writing there was an immediate increase in feelings of sadness and anxiety. However, in the long-term, compared to the control group, those who wrote about the emotionally charged topics had half the number of illness-related visits to the health center during the six months after the study. They also reported a greater sense of value and meaning as a result of the writing.

A subsequent study used the same protocol to assess the impact of expressive writing on the immune system by directly measuring immune markers in the blood. Results showed that the individuals who wrote about upsetting or traumatic experiences evidenced enhanced immune function compared to the control group. As in the previous study, they also experienced fewer health center visits.

In another early study, people who had been laid off from their jobs were asked to use expressive writing to describe their feelings about the lay-off for five consecutive days for 30 minutes. The results were notable: after three months, 27 percent of the participants landed jobs compared to just five percent in the control group, and seven months after writing, 53 percent had jobs compared to only 18 percent in the control group. Interestingly, both groups went to exactly the same number of job interviews. The researchers speculated that it was likely that the people who'd written about their emotions had more quickly come to terms with their anger about being laid off and had possibly come off as less hostile in interviews.

Since these initial studies, numerous other researchers have looked at the effect of expressive writing on many different populations. The evidence continues to show a profound impact on people's lives. What's more, writing does not just make people *feel* better, it results in measurable improvements in physical health. Using approaches similar to the studies described above, researchers have found that:

- People with asthma experienced improvements in lung function.
- People with arthritis experienced improvements in joint health, and the majority reported meaningful improvements in quality of life similar to those that would be expected from a successful drug treatment.
- People with arthritis and lupus reported less fatigue.
- For people with fibromyalgia, several studies have shown improvements in reducing symptoms and increasing quality of life.
- People with irritable bowel syndrome (IBS) reported a reduction in the severity of their symptoms.
- People living with HIV experienced enhanced immune function, including increased CD4 levels and lower viral load.
- People who had suffered a heart attack had fewer medical appointments, used fewer medications, were more engaged in self-care activities, and generally were doing better, including having lower blood pressure.

Expressive writing has also been shown to help wounds heal faster, to help people stop smoking, and to promote improved sleep. And while writing had no impact on the actual progression of the disease for people with cancer, it was shown to improve their ability to cope with the disease (particularly for people who were socially isolated).

Other studies of expressive writing interventions have looked at its potential to improve various measures relating to quality of life. In one study of married couples, participants who wrote about their marital problems experienced improvements in their relationships compared to a control group. In another study, expressive writing was shown to improve the college grades of freshmen African American students. Other research found that it reduced stigma-related stress among gay men. It has also been shown to benefit chronically stressed caregivers of older adults.

What seems especially notable is that there appear to be few groups of people, health conditions or aspects of life quality that do not benefit from the use of expressive writing.

The Reasons Behind Writing's Positive Impacts

<u>Translating Emotion into Language</u>
Many times, I've heard the participants in my workshops talk about the relief of getting an experience that was bothering them "out of my head and onto the page." I've had the same experience myself. There's something about translating feelings and experiences into written language that somehow loosens their hold on us and makes us feel better. But why is this?

Understanding how the brain works may provide at least part of the answer. A 2007 study conducted by Matthew D. Lieberman, a professor of psychology at UCLA, used brain imaging to understand why putting our feelings into words makes those feelings less intense. The study found that when participants were shown photographs of an angry or fearful face, they experienced increased activity in a region of the brain called the amygdala, which activates various biological responses that the body uses when it experiences danger.

Lieberman's study showed that when participants used language to describe the emotion they perceived in the photographs, the amygdala was less active while another region of the brain, the right ventrolateral prefrontal cortex, became more active. This part of the brain is involved in processing emotions and inhibiting behavior. Using language turns on this part of the brain, facilitating the brain's ability to manage our emotional states.

Writing about an emotion or an experience means that we can integrate it and move on. We no longer take up mental space processing it. We ruminate less. This supports better sleep and improved health markers.

You might wonder, if this is true, why not just talk about something rather write about it? The fact is that, unlike talking, writing is a solitary experience. When writing, you don't have to shape a narrative for anyone else or censor yourself. What's more, writing allows us to bypass our rational mind and access a more emotional, intuitive and associative self. I've lost count of the times in my workshops and classes when participants declared, "I had no idea I felt that way until I wrote about it!"

As a result, writing can bring to light the feelings that have been lurking under the surface. It allows us to process those feelings and understand them. With that understanding, we can make new choices in our lives.

Disclosing Secrets

In their book, *Opening Up by Writing It Down*, Pennebaker and Smyth speculate that because keeping secrets is a stressor on the body, writing things down reduces our stress. "Keeping back thoughts, feelings and behaviors," they say, "can place us at risk for major and minor diseases." In discussing this, they talk about how lie detector machines (polygraphs) track biological stress indicators. When someone tells a lie, they are withholding a secret and this shows up in increased pulse, blood pressure, perspiration, and rates of breathing, which are tracked by the polygraph.

Pennebaker and Smyth suggest that the traumatic or difficult experiences that we don't talk about create this kind of reaction on the body. In holding on to such an experience without discussing it, our bodily stress reactions may not be as dramatic as those that show up on a polygraph machine, but in the long term, they have definite negative impacts on our health.

Interestingly, Pennebaker and Smyth talk about how polygraphers (the experts who administer polygraph tests) have observed that in instances when people ended up confessing to a crime, their biological stress markers immediately go down. This is surprising since in many cases these people are likely facing negative serious negative consequences such as going to prison. This does seem to indicate that divulging secrets makes us feel better, even in cases where we might least expect it.

Most of us are unlikely to be covering up a serious crime, but we may be withholding the truth in other ways. Perhaps we've experienced a trauma or a loss that we haven't really talked about because of shame or simply because we don't want to burden others. Or perhaps we don't discuss feelings that we feel guilty about, such as resentment at having to care for an ill spouse or a disabled child. Or maybe we haven't fully expressed the feelings we have about experiences of social stigma or oppression, such as homophobia, racism, or sexism.

Writing as Problem-Solving

Writing about an experience or feeling that we've kept hidden not only lessens physical stressors, but it also supports our ability to resolve our problems. As we write about experiences, we go through a process of remembering, understanding and making sense of them. Often, by making sense of a difficult experience, we can assign it new meaning. I've seen this happen particularly powerfully when people have recalled events that happened in childhood.

For example, a woman in one of my workshops had been bullied repeatedly by an older boy in her neighborhood when she was between the ages of seven and ten. At the time, she believed she deserved the bullying because, as an overweight girl, she got the message from many people in her life that being overweight meant she was lazy, greedy and unworthy. After writing as an adult about the experience of being bullied and what it meant to her, she came to a new understanding—she had not deserved it and the adults around her had failed her by not stopping it. From the writing, she was also able to see herself in a different light. She realized that her early experience had made her strong and resilient, and it had also made her deeply empathetic—she was often the first to speak out when she saw someone else being treated unfairly. Through her writing, she came to a new appreciation of herself and her strengths.

I've witnessed this kind of new self-understanding result from writing among many of my workshop participants. It's also something that's supported by the research. For example, Pennebaker and Smyth discuss how 70 percent of people who wrote about a trauma reported several months later that it helped them understand themselves and the event better. Pennebaker and Smyth suggest that writing about a traumatic event several times allows us to become more and more detached from the event itself. As a result, we can stand back and consider the complexity surrounding it and our own reactions. It means we can "see the bigger picture" and look at ourselves from a different, more neutral perspective. Often, this allows us to be more compassionate and understanding towards ourselves.

As a result, we can go from "I was bullied because I was a fat kid and I still feel ashamed," to "I didn't deserve to be bullied, but that experience made me a strong person who stands up for others."

The same principle can also apply to more small scale, everyday issues. For example, "I must be lazy because my boss is unhappy with my output this week," can become "I've had so many stresses this week that I just haven't been able to concentrate at work. I'll rest this weekend so I can focus more next week." In this way, writing allows us to reframe our experiences, and a problem that causes us worry or anxiety can become more manageable. And, because we feel we have resolved a problem—or at least found a solution we can execute—it no longer weighs so heavily on our minds.

In some cases (such as the laid-off workers or the married couples mentioned earlier who wrote about their feelings), writing about uncomfortable emotions such as anger, sadness or fear lessens the hold of those emotions on us. This means we're less likely to act them out and can result in a better performance in a job interview or make us less likely to pick a fight with our spouse.

Writing as Empowerment

Beyond its health benefits, writing is an amazing tool for self-development and self-understanding. It offers a potent means to explore our own thoughts and feelings. And writing down our thoughts and ideas puts us in touch with our own thinking potential—something that gives us a greater sense of empowerment in our lives. We are much less likely to think of ourselves as powerless if we experience ourselves as people who can articulate our problems, think them through, and find solutions for ourselves. In some cases, we can use the insights we gain from writing to make conscious positive changes in our lives.

I've seen this happen among many participants in my workshops. For example, a man who, through writing about his frustration with his teenage daughter, recognized that he was repeating the same angry and distancing patterns his own father had showed with him when he was a child. This allowed him to make a choice to change the way he was behaving and take responsibility for creating a better relationship with his daughter.

Writing as a Place for Calm

Finally, in a world filled with information overload and multiple distractions, writing can be a place where we find calm. Writing is the slowest of all uses of language and by stopping to write in a journal, for example, we slow down our minds. So many of us engage in social media and spend many hours on the internet each day. A recent study revealed that Americans check their phone on average once every 12 minutes, which works out to 80 times a day!

Many of these habits have been connected to increased anxiety and depression. Expressive writing can offer a simple antidote to this. It offers a place where, instead of reacting to an external barrage of information by liking, loving, clicking, or sharing, we focus on our own thoughts and feelings and connect with the things that really matter to us. Instead of following what's trending on Twitter, we check in with what's happening with ourselves. I can't help believing that this kind of practice makes us happier and healthier human beings equipped to live more satisfying lives.

14

CHAPTER TWO
HOW TO APPROACH THE WRITING EXERCISES

"Writing practice brings us back to the uniqueness of our own minds and an acceptance of it. We all have wild dreams, fantasies, and ordinary thoughts. Let us to feel the texture of them and not be afraid of them."
Natalie Goldberg, *Wild Mind: Living the Writer's Life*

What Gets in the Way

As we've already established, writing is a powerful tool to support your health and happiness. However, to get the full benefit that writing offers, it's important that you approach it in a particular way. And because this may not be the way that you generally approach writing, I want to briefly discuss what you need to do to get the most out of the exercises in this book.

It's not unusual for people to have negative associations with writing. Most of us learn to write at school where our efforts are constantly judged and graded. Throughout our lives, writing is usually seen as something that we do for others—teachers, professors, employers, or the "friends" in our social media feeds. And writing is generally done for external motives—to get good grades, to appear witty or intelligent, to impress a supervisor, to get a job. It's seldom seen as a tool for true self-expression. For this reason alone, it's common for people to feel uncomfortable using writing to explore their experiences and to express their feelings and thoughts.

In school, some of us took easily to learning the rules of spelling, grammar and syntax, others may have found these things illusive or challenging. If we were made to feel self-conscious about our difficulties in these areas, it makes sense that we become self-conscious when we write.

We also live in a society that doesn't tend to value the experiences of ordinary individuals. Our culture pays attention to the rich, famous, and powerful, but makes little room for the voices of regular people. The experiences and opinions of oppressed groups are even further discounted. If you're a woman, a person of color, a person with a disability, or a member of the LGBTQ community, for example, you've likely received a lot of subtle and not-so-subtle messages that your opinion or experience isn't valued by the mainstream culture. It's hard not to internalize those messages.

Regardless of our position in society, many of us have developed a harsh inner critic. It's the internal voice that judges every word we write and demands perfection of every sentence. It might constantly murmur, "Why are you writing? You have nothing worthwhile to say!" or, "What a terrible sentence! You need to erase that!" every time you put something on the page. Most participants in my workshops have some version of this voice.

That inner critic may resemble the voice of a parent or a teacher, or it might just be an amalgam of all the judgments that you've felt from people you know and the wider culture. In an odd way, that critical voice is trying to help us. By preventing us from speaking up or revealing our feelings, it's seeking to protect us from external judgment, criticism, embarrassment, or shame. Instead, though, by silencing us and stuffing our emotions, it ends up doing us harm.

I also see people bring a lot of judgment of the feelings and thoughts that show up on the page. "I hate that I'm so negative!" I might hear one of my workshop participants declare. Someone else might say, "Why do I sound so angry?" or, "Why do I keep writing about the same experience again and again?" It's important to remember that it's very normal to have negative feelings or thoughts. There's nothing inherently wrong with being angry or sad. In fact, these and other challenging emotions are what make us human and, as noted in the previous chapter, suppressing them can have harmful effects on our health.

If you find yourself revisiting the same themes, feelings or experiences in your writing, that simply means you still need to process them. It takes time to express, understand, and metabolize the full complexity of some things that have happened to us. Don't judge yourself for it, simply write about those things for as long as you need.

Guidelines for the Exercises

Because so many of us have barriers or fears about writing, I've put together these guidelines for how to get the most out of the exercises in this book. Please follow them as closely as you can.

1. When you write, don't worry about spelling, punctuation, grammar or syntax. And don't concern yourself with style or tone, or even whether what you're writing makes a lot of sense. Instead, focus on connecting with yourself, your thoughts and feelings. Write whatever comes into your mind.

2. Try as best you can to let go of all the judgments and criticism you bring to your writing and to yourself. If you notice your inner critic showing up, ask it gently to take a break.

3. Try to write without pausing and without thinking too much about what you're putting on the page. The idea is that you write in a way that circumvents your left-brain, logical filters and instead connect with your right-brain intuitive, creative self. This intuitive self allows us access to our emotions and can provide insights that are not available to us when we remain stuck in our rational mind.

4. While it's possible to write anywhere at any time, it can help to set aside a quiet time and place. Try to find somewhere that's comfortable and where you won't be distracted. Let the people around you know you don't want to be interrupted. Turn off your cellphone or put it in another room.

5. To connect with your innermost thoughts and feelings, it can help to get yourself in a calm and centered space before you write. At the end of this chapter, I provide a centering exercise you can use before you begin writing. While using this technique isn't necessary, you may find it helpful.

How to Use the Exercises

The writing exercises in this book have been thoughtfully designed to address different aspects of wellness. I've created these exercises based upon the following things:

1. The evidence showing what works when it comes to using writing as a wellness tool.

2. My own extensive experience of facilitating workshops and classes in a variety of settings.

3. Techniques I've used with success in my coaching practice to help clients connect with their deepest selves, overcome limiting beliefs, and adopt healthy behaviors.

Be aware that you can do the exercises once, or you can do them many times. In fact, there's no limit on how many times you can repeat the exercises in a specific chapter, and doing so is something you may want to consider. This is simply because the more you write, the more connected you become to your intuitive self and the remarkable wisdom it holds.

Managing Feelings

Some of the exercises in this book invite you to explore negative experiences or emotions. When writing about these things, it's only natural and normal that you may have difficult or uncomfortable feelings arise. If this happens, please bear the following things in mind:

1. Many of us are taught to be uncomfortable about expressing any kinds of emotions, particularly "negative" emotions like sadness or anger. American culture is particularly forceful in telling people that it's important to remain "positive" and "upbeat." But all of us feel sad or angry at some time. Putting these feelings down on paper doesn't make these emotions any bigger and, in most cases, writing about them will help loosen their hold on you.

2. If you find that writing brings up traumatic memories or feelings you find hard to manage, it's important that you pay attention to how much they are upsetting you. You may simply feel better a day or two after writing about these things. Or it could be that you just need to step back and take a break from writing. Perhaps you need to engage in a lot of self-care. You may also want to consider talking to someone you trust about how you're feeling—for example, a supportive friend, partner or spouse.

3. If the emotions that get churned up start to feel difficult for you to manage, you may want to consider seeking out a peer support group or professional help. We're most likely to feel this way when writing about past trauma, or recent and past grief and loss.

   While confiding our feelings to the page can be immensely helpful and healing, it's important to recognize that you do not have to deal with your feelings alone. You could start by talking with your doctor, or reach out to a counselor or a therapist, or look up what kind of other resources there might be for people who have had similar experiences to you. There are many people with the desire and expertise to help you.

Writing in Groups

Another thing to consider is using this book with a group of other people. These may be individuals who share the same challenges that you're experiencing—perhaps the recent loss of a loved one or difficulty dealing with a debilitating health condition. Or you might just want to gather a group of friends who want to come together to write on the different wellness themes dealt with in the various chapters, or to use writing for self-development.

Writing with a group of others helps create social connection and a sense of community. It can be also a place where you share excerpts of what you write. This can help lessen feelings of isolation and offer support when you are going through difficult experiences. If you are interested in forming a wellness writing group, make sure to look at the detailed guidelines I provide on this in Chapter Ten.

Centering Exercise

One major reason that writing is such an effective tool in promoting health and wellness is that it allows us to access our unconscious. While some people may be able to jump right into a writing exercise and easily connect to the more intuitive part of our minds, others may find it more challenging.

One way of making it easier to access that part of ourselves through writing is to do a short centering exercise prior to starting. It will help get you into a more relaxed mental state. This kind of centering can be especially helpful when you're first starting out and not yet used to writing down your innermost feelings and thoughts. It can also be particularly helpful if you find that your mind is racing or you're especially anxious or agitated.

Here are the instructions:

Find a place where you can feel relaxed and remain without interruption for at least five minutes. Get into a comfortable position. You can sit on a chair, cross-legged (or otherwise) on the ground, or you can lie down. Close your eyes and take six long, deep breaths. As you do so, notice where you are holding tension in your body. This might be in your neck and shoulders, in your back, your hips and pelvis, or any other part of your body. As you notice the tension, try to relax those muscles. Imagine that any stress or tension is sinking away and falling into the earth. Simply let all of it drop from your body and into the ground.

Continue to breathe slowly and evenly for the next two or three minutes. As you do so, try to focus your mind on the gentle in and out motion of your breath. If your mind wanders, that's fine, but when you notice it, bring your attention back to your breath.

You can take as long as you want to do this exercise, but I would suggest a minimum of five minutes. If you want, you can set a timer for the desired amount to time you want to spend. Once you are done, open your notebook or your computer and start the exercise or journal entry you want to write.

If you find it difficult to do this exercise without additional guidance, there are many apps, CDs or downloadable audio resources that provide brief guided meditations that you can use.

CHAPTER THREE
WRITE FOR OVERALL HEALTH AND WELLNESS

"Writing, like all arts, can aid healing because people who understand their wants and needs, or hopes and fears, better are less likely to become ill, experience less severe symptoms when they do, and tend to recover more quickly, or are more at peace with chronic or terminal illness."

Gillian Bolton, *Write Yourself: Creative Writing and Personal Development*

As I described earlier, writing can be used by anyone as a tool to support overall wellness, regardless of background, life situation or health status. In this chapter, I outline a variety of techniques and exercises you can use with this goal in mind.

Keep a Journal

One very simple way to help improve your overall wellness is to keep a journal. A journal allows you to record experiences, explore feelings, and come to a new understanding of events in your life. In keeping your journal, bear in mind the guidelines for writing in Chapter Two—don't censor yourself, don't worry about spelling or grammar, put your inner critic aside. Treat it as a place where you can confide your deepest secrets. This may require that you store it in a secure place or, if it's on a computer, make sure it's password-protected. Do whatever you need to do so you're not afraid that someone else will read what you have written without your permission.

You can keep your journal in a notebook or on your computer or tablet. However, if you are going to use an electronic device, I strongly suggest that, while you write, you turn off any notifications that will distract you. To get the most benefit from journal writing, do it in a place where you're relaxed and won't be interrupted. It's also good to assign a regular time to do it, because this helps create a regular habit that you'll stick to. Many people write in their journals first thing in the morning, the idea being that immediately after sleep (when our unconscious mind has been at its most active) we can more easily access our creativity and intuition. Journal writing first thing in the morning can also establish a foundational habit that can help us stick to our desired routines, goals and activities throughout the day.

For some people, writing early in the morning may just not be possible. Another good time to journal can also be in the evening, when you have a chance to reflect on your day. Again, this may not be possible for everyone and you may find that the best time for you to write is during your lunchtime or a break.

If possible, try to take at least 20 minutes to write. If you want to, write for longer. But try to get in the habit of putting at least 20 minutes aside. However, if you can only grab 10 minutes, that also works.

If you haven't kept a journal before, you may wonder what you should write about. The answer is whatever you want. But if it's challenging to know where to start, here are some suggestions:

- Write about things that you most enjoyed today.
- Write about an experience that touched you.
- Write about what challenged or frustrated you.
- Write about a moment in your day that made you feel a strong emotion (for example, happy, angry, sad, shocked, resentful, outraged, appreciative).
- Write about an event from your day that made an impression on you.
- Write about something that puzzled or confused you.
- Write about something you did today that made you feel good about yourself.
- Write about something that happened that made you feel good towards another person.
- Write about something you feel guilty for.
- Write about something that made you feel relaxed and calm.
- Write about something that gave you joy.
- Write about something you are grateful for.

When you use one of these prompts, you may find that your writing veers off in unexpected directions or you may find yourself writing about a feeling, memory or experience that you hadn't anticipated. That's good. This is because if you surprise yourself with where you're writing goes, then you're accessing that less rational/logical part of your mind. That part of your mind puts you in touch with your deeper self, accesses emotion and intuition, and allows you to engage in creative problem-solving.

Keep a Gratitude Journal

Several studies have indicated that keeping a gratitude journal can have positive impacts on people's health and outlook. For example, in one study, people with neuromuscular disorders were asked to make lists each night before sleeping of things for which they were grateful. After three weeks of maintaining this habit, participants reported getting longer and more refreshing sleep.

Another study published in *Psychosomatic Medicine* in 2016 examined the impact of keeping a gratitude journal among people with Stage B heart failure. Half of the study participants were randomly assigned to keep a daily gratitude journal, in which they were asked to record three to five things for which they were grateful each day. This group showed greater signs of improved heart health (such as reduced inflammation and increased heart rate variability), compared to the group that didn't journal.

Other studies have shown that feeling and expressing gratitude creates a positive attitude, reduces worry and rumination, and increases life satisfaction and optimism. Keeping a regular gratitude journal keeps us in touch with all the things we appreciate in our lives and directs our focus away from the things that may irk or worry us. Research suggests that writing your gratitude journal at the end of the day can have the added benefit of reducing insomnia and enhancing overall sleep quality.

You can keep a gratitude journal by writing about the things you are grateful for each day. This can be a very simple list, or you can choose to write at greater length. For example, you might just write, "I'm grateful for the way that my boss listened to me today," or you may describe in more detail why this was important and what it meant to you.

Beyond detailing what you're grateful for in your day, you can also choose to use your gratitude journal for other positive aspects of your life. The following are a list of prompts that you can use to get you started:

- Write about a skill or talent that you are grateful that you have.
- Write about a person you're especially grateful for and why.
- How has your life changed in positive ways over the last year?
- What activities and hobbies do you especially enjoy? Write about them and how you feel when doing them.
- List a part of your body that you're grateful for and why.
- What comforts in your life do you especially appreciate?

- Write what you love about art and the role it plays in your life.
- Write what you love about music and the role it plays in your life.
- Write about what you love about nature.
- What have you enjoyed learning this week?
- Describe in detail a meal you particularly enjoyed this week.
- What do you look forward to when you wake in the morning?
- Write a letter to someone who had a positive impact on your life.
- When was the last time you laughed uncontrollably? Write about it.
- Write about how you helped someone this week.
- Describe a moment of connection with someone (it can be a loved one, a co-worker or a stranger) that really improved your day.
- Write about a talent or skill that you used today.

Writing Exercises to Support Wellness

The following exercises are support overall wellness and are based on research-derived evidence.

Imagine Your Best Self

Envisioning a future "best self" and writing about that self has been shown to have long-term positive impacts on people's health.

The following exercise should be done over five days. It's best if you do it over four consecutive days, but if that's not possible, try to do it over no more than 10 days. On days one to three, you'll need no more than 20 minutes. Day four will require about 40 minutes to an hour.

Day One: Imagine yourself one year from now. Imagine that you are your best possible self. Write about who you are, what you are doing, your relationships, what you have achieved. Write about this in detail for at least 20 minutes.

Day Two: Imagine yourself in five years. Imagine that you are your best possible self. Write about who you are, what you are doing, your relationships, what you have achieved. Write about this in detail for at least 20 minutes.

Day Three: Imagine yourself in 10 years. Imagine that you are your best possible self. Write about who you are, what you are doing, your relationships, what you have achieved. Write about this in detail for at least 20 minutes.

Day Four: Read over what you've written on each of the previous days. Read slowly and thoughtfully. Once you've finished, spend a little time thinking about all the positive qualities and assets you see in your "best future self."

Now spend 20 minutes writing about what you would like to do over the next three to six months so you can become that "best future self."

Nurture a Positive Relationship with Your Body

We live in a culture that tends to encourage us to focus on what's wrong with our bodies. Women, especially, are taught to try to fit some unattainable ideal. Those of us who don't fit society's notion of perfect fitness, beauty, health, or appearance find it particularly challenging to love and appreciate our physical selves.

One way we can cultivate a healthier self-image is to build a positive relationship with the body that we have. The following exercises can help you do just that. They are designed to be done over a few days. In responding to them, write whatever comes into your mind and try not to censor yourself.

Day One: Write about the first time you remember being self-conscious or ashamed about your body. Describe the experience, what happened, and how it made you feel. Write for at least 20 minutes.

Day Two: Think about all the messages that you get now that make you feel physically inadequate, self-conscious or ashamed. Write about them and write about how they make you feel. Write for at least 20 minutes.

Day Three: Write about doing something physical that you enjoy a lot. It can be dancing, walking, running, swimming, wading in the ocean, a sport, a game, tending your garden. Try to describe in great detail your physical sensations and emotions when you do this. Write for at least 20 minutes.

Day Four: Write about what you love or like about your body. It might be a particular body part, a physical talent, or how your body responds to a sexual or sensual experience. Write for at least 20 minutes.

Day Five: Imagine your body has a voice. Write that voice. Let your body express itself freely in words. Write for at least 20 minutes.

Day Six: Having completed the exercises above, spend some time reading over them. After that, spend 20 to 45 minutes writing about what you've learned about how you feel about your body and what you'd like to change about how you relate to and treat your body.

The series of six exercises above can be done more than once. You may want to try doing these six exercises and then, after working to implement the changes that you've decide to make in the final exercise, repeat the series of exercises again. You will likely find that doing this will provide new and potentially deeper insights and will help you decrease any negative self-talk and criticism you have about your body and yourself overall.

Become a Better Problem-Solver

All of us face problems and obstacles. They can be in relationships with partners, spouses, children, friends, or family members. They might concern work or money. Or they might be internal obstacles we just don't seem able to resolve. Often, we find ourselves worrying about these issues. While we ruminate, we might find ourselves distracted at work, unable to pay attention to our families, or unable to sleep at night.

Writing has been shown to help people become better problem solvers. In part, this is because getting our concerns down on paper helps us clarify them (it also helps us stop worrying and promotes better sleep, which, in turn, can improve our thinking). Writing can also allow us to access our intuition and creativity, thus providing insights that our logical mind might not have.

The exercise below helps you clarify any problem and gain insight into how to solve it. You can do it in one sitting (which should take from 30 minutes to an hour). However, each section of the exercise can also be done in three separate sittings of 10 to 20 minutes each.

Step One. Write about a problem you are facing. Write about it in detail. Don't censor your thoughts and feelings, just focus on getting the words down on the page. Write for 10 to 20 minutes.

Step Two: Spend a few minutes reading over what you've written. Once you've finished reading, take a couple of minutes to sit quietly and reflect on what you read and try to identify the key barriers or issues in this problem. Try to focus on the aspects of the issue that you have control of or can change. Now write about these issues for 10 to 20 minutes.

Step Three: Reread what you wrote in step one and two. Take a couple of minutes to sit quietly and reflect on what you read. Now write for 10 to 20 minutes, focusing on your thoughts and insights about the problem, barriers to overcoming it, and identify potential solutions.

Create an Inner Mentor

Sometimes we may find ourselves making decisions that later, with the benefit of hindsight, we realize were not in our best interests. This could be anything from taking a job that we *knew* was not the right fit even during the interview, to agreeing to a date with someone who strikes us as a little "off," to buying a car or other item that was beyond our budget. We all know the feeling of regret and frustration that comes from not trusting our intuition or the wiser self that told us to not take the job, go on the date, or buy the car.

In this exercise, you will create an inner mentor or higher self who you can access on those moments when you need to make a decision. Once you have created this inner mentor, you can rely on this mentor for wisdom and help whenever you need it.

Step One: Think back to a time in your life when there was a person who acted as a mentor, teacher or role model. This should be someone who consistently had your best interests at heart. Write about that person and all the qualities that you admired and that helped you. Write for 10 to 20 minutes. (If you had the misfortune of never having such a person in your life, write instead about your "ideal mentor," the person you wished you had in your life when you needed someone like that. If you want, give that ideal mentor a name.)

Step Two: Read over what you wrote about your real or ideal mentor. Now, write about all the ways that this mentor can help you going forward in your life. Ask that mentor to stay with you and be present whenever you need to ask them to help you out. Write for 10 to 20 minutes.

Step Three: Now you have your mentor, feel free to ask them for help whenever you are facing a challenging decision. When you need their help, write out your problem, then write out the advice that they offer you. Write for as long as you need.

Reduce Your Stress

There's no doubt among researchers and medical practitioners that long-term stress has negative impacts on our health. There's also compelling evidence to suggest that expressive writing can help reduce your stress levels.

If you are bothered by ongoing stress or if there is an issue or problem that is weighing on your mind, then you may want to try using the following exercises, which are modeled on exercises shown in several studies to reduce stress and improve other health markers.

Stress Reduction Exercise One:

Think of a topic that is bothering you. It might be something that you have not disclosed or discussed with anyone else. Without censoring yourself or editing your words, write about this topic for 20 to 30 minutes.

Once you have finished writing, review what you've written. Pay attention to how you feel and ask yourself if you have any new insights. If so, write these down.

You'll achieve the best results if you repeat this exercise over the course of three to five days. This will allow you to deepen your understanding of the problem, explore creative solutions, and to develop more compassion for yourself. Many people report that after doing this exercise for a few days in a row, they are able to either solve the problem or significantly reduce its impact on them.

Stress Reduction Exercise Two:

Day One: Think about the word stress. Write everything you can think of that's associated with this word for you. Write for about 20 minutes, without censoring or editing yourself.

Day Two: Review what you wrote. Are there themes or topics that stand out to you? If so, pick the theme or topic that has the most charge for you. Write about it for about 20 minutes.

Day Three: Review what you wrote on day one and two. Pay attention to any patterns that you notice or any new revelations. Write about what you think you can change or do differently that would help you deal with your stress. Write for 20 minutes.

You can repeat the exercise several times, or use it whenever you find yourself worrying or feeling stressed out. It's also possible to do the writing exercises for all three days in one sitting. However, if you leave some time between writing and reading what you've written, it may provide some emotional distance and help you come up with new insights.

Resolve Internal Conflict

Humans are complicated, it's part of our nature. Often, this means we are at odds with ourselves internally. For example, we may believe that we want to give up smoking or start eating healthier foods, but then we end up buying another pack of cigarettes or scarfing down a couple of donuts for breakfast. This kind of pattern can result in self-sabotage and seriously undermine our health. One way to begin to shift these patterns is to bring our awareness to them and understand the dynamics behind them. This exercise helps you with that process. You can do the three steps in one sitting, or you can do them over three days. Total time of the exercise is 30 minutes to an hour.

Step One: Visualize the part of you that undermines or sabotages your healthy intentions. It might be that part of you that overrides your plan to get to bed at a decent hour or that decides to remain on the couch when you'd planned to take a walk. Give that part of you a voice. Write what it has to say. (It's important when you do this to not censor or judge what that part of you has to say, simply let your writing give it a voice.) Write for 10 to 20 minutes.

Step Two: Now visualize the part of your that wants to put your health and well-being first. Give that part of you a voice. Write what it has to say. (When you do this, don't focus on responding negatively to what you wrote in step one, simply give voice to the part of you that wants to be healthy.) Write for 10 to 20 minutes.

Step Three: Review what you wrote in steps one and two. Think about what it would take for the two parts of you to come to an agreement that each of them can be happy about. (Such an agreement could involve compromises, resolving to be kinder and more empathetic to your "unhealthy" self, and creating realistic expectations.) Write out the agreement between the two parts of yourself. Write for 10 to 20 minutes.

Elaine Beale

CHAPTER FOUR
WRITE TO MANAGE CHRONIC ILLNESS AND PAIN

"Several very high quality studies have shown that expressive writing, added to standard medical treatment/care, can improve serious medical illnesses including asthma, arthritis, HIV/AIDS, and PTSD. Writing can help people dealing with chronic medical conditions, either at diagnosis or in the ongoing management of chronic or progressive illness, including cancers and possibly cardiovascular disease."

James W. Pennebaker, PhD and Joshua M. Smyth, PhD., *Opening Up by Writing It Down.*

Having a chronic health condition can be painful and isolating. It can make your life financially precarious. It may mean you have to depend on others for care. And while healthy people can take certain things for granted, having a chronic health condition can make many areas of your life feel out of your control.

What makes things worse is that we live in a society that often measures people's worth by how hard they work and how much they produce. The busier you are, the better you are. If you're sick, you're often seen as a shirker. Sometimes, you're treated as if being ill is your fault. Mainstream medicine frequently judges people negatively for having health conditions associated with being overweight or related to addictions like smoking. Alternative practitioners and gurus sometimes imply that people are to blame for their illnesses, suggesting, for example, that negative attitudes result in diseases like cancer.

There's no wonder that people often experience shame and self-blame for having a chronic health condition. We might ask ourselves, "What did I do to cause this?" or take our illness as an indication that we are worthless or bad. This only adds to our suffering. And, while there may be things we can do to take better care of ourselves and alleviate our symptoms, we're far less likely to engage in self-care if we burden ourselves with self-hatred or shame.

Numerous studies have shown that expressive writing can help improve the symptoms of people with an array of chronic health conditions—among them, fibromyalgia, arthritis, lupus, IBS, and hypertension. It has also been shown to improve immune function in people living with HIV, to help wounds heal faster, and help people with cancer cope with their disease.

People living with chronic illness or pain can certainly benefit from any of the exercises and techniques outlined in Chapter Three. And because many people with chronic illnesses do not have the emotional outlets that others may find at work in other relationships outside the home, keeping a journal can be especially helpful. Writing might not make up for a lack of social interaction, but confiding your feelings to the page can help immensely when there's no listening ear.

Journaling to Help Manage Chronic Illness and Pain
A gratitude journal (described in Chapter Three), can be especially useful since it's easy to dwell on what's wrong or be overwhelmed by negative feelings when dealing with a chronic illness or pain. Cultivating gratitude can help us remember the things we enjoy or appreciate. What's more, recent discoveries in neuroscience reveal that chronic pain results from altered circuits in the brain. This then leads to altered emotional and cognitive responses, creating a negative feedback loop in which the brain is unable to regulate pain as it normally would. Writing can be one tool that interrupts this process by getting us to focus on the positive, such as what we appreciate in life.

Because focusing on our pain or symptoms can potentially reinforce or exacerbate them, it's a good idea not to use a journal to simply ruminate on these things. However, a journal can be useful as a tool to help you tune in to your body so you make sure you don't push yourself too far physically, exacerbate symptoms, and to identify ways in which you might soothe, comfort, or care for yourself. Prompts that might be useful include the following:

- Today my body needs….
- I will care for myself today by….
- Today, being kind to myself means that I will…

- Today I will give myself pleasure by….
- Today I will not pay attention to "should," instead, I will…
- I am not defined by my illness. Instead, I am…
- If I were my own best friend today, I would….
- Describe in detail one thing you will do for yourself today that will provide you comfort.
- Make a list of all the things that made you feel appreciative or joyful over the last week.

Exercises to Help Manage Chronic Illness and Pain

The exercises below are designed for individuals who have a chronic health condition to increase self-compassion and understanding, decrease stress, nurture a positive mindset, and support improved long-term health outcomes.

Exercise: Understanding How We Relate to Our Illness

Often, our attitude to illness and toward ourselves when we are sick may get in the way of taking care of ourselves and cultivating self-compassion. These attitudes were often learned earlier in life. The following series of exercises help us uncover the attitudes towards illness that we learned in childhood and adolescence and reflect on them. This can help reduce negative self-talk and improve how we treat ourselves. It's best if you do the exercises over a series of six days so that you are more able to reflect on what you've written. But you can also do the exercises in one sitting if you'd prefer. Total time is between one to two hours. As you write, remember to not censor or edit yourself and just write what comes into your head.

Step One: Write about a time you were sick as a child. Remember how you felt and how your parents or other caregivers treated you. Write about it in as much detail as you can. Write for 10 to 20 minutes.

Step Two: Write about all the things you learned about illness as a child, a teenager, and as a young adult. Write for 10 to 20 minutes.

Step Three: Perhaps you had family members who were ill. Or perhaps everyone was robustly healthy. We learn from our family's attitudes and actions around illness. Write about illness in your family. Write for 10 to 20 minutes.

Step Four: Write about what you learned about medicine and doctors as a child, teen and young adult. Write for 10 to 20 minutes.

Step Five: Read over what you wrote in response to this exercise over the last four days. Think about what this writing says about what you learned about illness and what being sick means to you now. Write about these things for 10 to 20 minutes.

Step Six: Now you've written about and reflected on your attitudes to illness, write about attitudes or behaviors you'd like to change. Pay attention to how you can increase your compassion for yourself and what you can do to better care for yourself. Write for 10 to 20 minutes.

Exercise: Coming to Terms with Illness

It can be challenging to come to terms with having a chronic health condition. It's completely natural to feel angry or resentful at how it restricts or changes your life. Sometimes we may turn that anger inward, berating or shaming ourselves. Sometimes, in our refusal to accept our body's limitations, we may try to ignore or fight our symptoms. This can result in us not taking caring of ourselves or pushing past our limits.

It's best if you do the exercises over five days so that you are more able to reflect on what you've written. But you can also do the exercises in one sitting if you'd prefer. Total time is between an hour and an hour and 40 minutes. As you write, remember to not censor or edit yourself and just write what comes into your head.

Step One: Write about when you first received your diagnosis or when you first became ill. Write for 10 to 20 minutes.

Step Two: Write about all the losses you've experienced because of your illness. Write for 10 to 20 minutes.

Step Three: Make a list of the negative things you tell yourself about being ill. Write for 10 to 20 minutes.

Step Four: Write about any positive things that have come out of being ill, or, write about what your illness has taught you. Write for 10 to 20 minutes.

Step Five: Read over everything you wrote in steps one through four above. Does this lead you to want to make any changes in your life? Write about what you've learned and what you'd like to do differently. Write for 10 to 20 minutes.

Exercise: Listen to Your Body

We live in a culture that doesn't really encourage us to pay deep attention to our bodies. As a result, we often don't really notice how we feel physically.

Instead, it's seen as virtuous to work through pain, to show up to your job when you're ill, or to "overcome" a disability rather than pay attention to and honor your physical limitations.

For people who are living with chronic illness, it's particularly important to pay attention to our physical needs since pushing through pain or ignoring symptoms can often make us feel far worse. The following brief exercise helps you tune into your body. You can use it once, but you can also use on an ongoing basis to help you pay closer attention to your body and its needs. You can do all three steps on consecutive days, or you can do them all in one sitting. Total time is between 30 minutes and an hour.

Step One: Imagine that your body has its own voice. Write what it wants to tell you. Write for 10 to 20 minutes.

Step Two: Read over what you wrote in step one. Now respond to your body. Write for 10 to 20 minutes.

Step Three: Reflect on what you just wrote in steps one and two. Now write about how you'd like to treat your body. This may involve changes in your behavior or perhaps paying closer attention to your body's signals. Write for 10 to 20 minutes.

Exercise: Talk to your illness

If you have a chronic illness or health condition, you have to decide how to manage it and also how you relate to it emotionally and mentally. This exercise helps you explore your options and potentially develop a more harmonious relationship with your illness or pain. You can do this exercise in one sitting or over two or three days. Total time is about an hour.

Step One: Imagine you are sitting in a room. Your chronic illness or condition has stepped out of your body and is sitting across from you. Write a conversation between you and your illness. Start by telling your illness/condition how you feel about it. Then let it respond. Write for 20 minutes.

Step Two: Read over what you wrote. Write about what you learned from this exercise? Write for 20 minutes.

Step Three: Make a list of any changes that you'd like to make in how you relate to your illness.

Exercise: Take better care of yourself

This exercise helps you explore your attitudes towards being ill and examine what you are doing to support or undermine your own health. It's best if you do the exercises over a series of four days so that you are more able to reflect on what you've written. But you can also do the exercises in one sitting if you'd prefer. Total time is between 40 minutes and one hour, 20 minutes.

Step One: Write about what it means to you to be ill. Write for 10 to 20 minutes.

Step Two: Think about all the ways that you undermine or don't take care of your health. Write about them. Write for 10 to 20 minutes.

Step Three: Think about all the ways that you do take care of yourself and support your health. Write about them. Write for 10 to 20 minutes.

Step Four: Review what you wrote in steps one through three. Now write about what changes you'd like to make in your attitudes or behaviors to take better care of yourself and your health. Write for 10 to 20 minutes.

Exercise: Lift Your Mood, Relieve Symptoms

Being sick or in pain is often accompanied by feelings of depression, sadness, frustration, or other negative emotions. This can further compound our suffering and make our symptoms feel worse. Research has shown that writing about positive experiences can lift mood and improve symptoms and pain. This exercise helps improve mood and potentially lessen our awareness of painful or difficult symptoms.

Choose from the following prompts to start your writing. You can use these prompts whenever you want to shift your attention to something positive and enjoyable. Write for as long as you want.

- Think about a time from your childhood when you were very happy. It might be a day at the beach, a birthday celebration, a shared moment with a friend, an achievement at school, or an afternoon spent in solitary play. Write about it in great detail. Try to bring in all your senses (sights, sounds, textures, tastes, smells).

- Think about a place you love and that you associate with relaxation or pleasure. Write about it in detail. Try to bring in all your senses.

- Think about a "peak experience" from your life. It might be falling in love, playing a sport that you love, visiting a beautiful place, or dancing all night. Write about it in detail. Try to bring in all your senses.

- Think about something that you enjoy doing so much that sometimes you get so absorbed in it you lose track of time. It might be a hobby, a sport, something creative, something physical. Write about that experience in detail. Try to bring in all your senses.

- Think about a person you love(d) deeply. It might be someone from your childhood, a partner, spouse, friend or family member. Write about that person, focusing on all the qualities in them that you love and the positive things that they have brought to you and your life.

CHAPTER FIVE
WRITE TO HEAL FROM TRAUMA

"The act of writing helps name the unnameable: the chaotic feelings we resist, fear or remain unaware of... your pain becomes manageable, explorable, transformable, into unexpected patterns of meaning."

Gabriele Rico, *Pain and Possibility: Writing Your Way Through Personal Crisis*

What is Trauma?

Trauma is defined as a psychological, emotional response to an event or experience that is deeply distressing or disturbing. This definition could apply to an upsetting event, such as losing a loved one, going through a divorce, or witnessing a car accident. However, it also encompasses more extreme experiences such as rape, violent assault, or fighting in a war.

Clearly, there are different levels of trauma and our responses to a particular traumatic experience are colored by our history, background, age, and access to safety and support. Typical initial reactions to a traumatic event are shock and denial. Long-term responses might include anger, persistent feelings of sadness and despair, unpredictable emotions, flashbacks, and feelings of isolation and hopelessness.

Survivors might also have physical symptoms, such as nausea and headaches, or they may experience guilt or shame, as if they are somehow responsible for the event. (Shame and guilt are often made worse by societal attitudes that, for example, blame women who were sexually assaulted for dressing "inappropriately" or somehow "asking for it." This and other forms of victim-blaming are pervasive and greatly exacerbate the suffering of survivors of many kinds of violence and abuse.)

While trauma can take a terrible toll on people, it's important to remember that not everyone is scarred by a traumatic experience, and some people are able to move on relatively quickly while others experiencing a similar event may take much longer to heal. This means that there is no "right way" to recover and the process is individual, so it's important not to judge yourself or compare yourself to others as you go through your own healing.

The Long-Term Health Costs of Trauma

Trauma can take an enormous toll on our well-being. It has been linked with depression and anxiety disorders as well as post-traumatic stress disorder (PTSD). In his pioneering book, *The Body Keeps the Score*, Bessel van der Kolk details how trauma results in damaging physiological changes to the body and brain that can predispose us to illness. He goes on to discuss how trauma can negatively impact relationships and families, and many other aspects of our lives.

Research indicates a stunning correlation between childhood trauma and poor physical health. For example, the groundbreaking Adverse Childhood Experiences Study (a long-term study conducted by Kaiser Permanente and the Centers for Disease Control) demonstrated that the higher the level of childhood trauma an individual experienced, the more likely he or she was to have heart disease, lung cancer, diabetes, and many autoimmune diseases, as well as depression and other mental illness. In fact, those individuals with six or more categories of abuse or dysfunction as children had a life expectancy 20 years lower than those with none.

While trauma's health impacts are potentially severe, it is possible for to heal. Numerous interventions have been shown to be effective in allowing people to recover and move on with their lives. As detailed in Chapter One, writing is one such tool for recovery. For some people, writing has been the central practice they've used to support their healing. Others have used it as an adjunct to therapy, peer support groups or other interventions.

Writing and Trauma

The way the brain works during trauma may provide the answer about why expressive writing can help in healing. The two sides of our brain process information differently. The left side is the rational brain, which recalls facts and includes the area responsible for speech, thus providing the words we use when we explain something that happened in a sequential order. During a traumatic situation, activity in the left brain decreases dramatically, explaining why rational speech is often difficult for trauma survivors. As Bessel van der Kolk notes, "All trauma is preverbal…. Our bodies re-experience terror, rage, helplessness, as well as the impulse to fight or flee, but these feelings are almost impossible to articulate."

Traumatized people may find it extremely difficult to talk about their experience even years afterwards. Van der Kolk points out that when people are able to talk about it, they often give the left brain version, that is, the rational mind's explanation of their symptoms and behaviors. This version does not involve the right brain's deeply felt emotions—which explains why people can sometimes speak about a terrible experience without any apparent emotion in their face or voice. Van der Kolk states that full healing only occurs when both sides of the brain are engaged.

As van der Kolk notes, journaling and writing is one way to engage both sides of the brain to help healing. By writing, we put words (left brain) to our sensations and feelings (right brain). This allows us to fully articulate our emotions and integrate the experience, making it possible for us to heal and move on.

A Word of Caution

While writing can be a potent tool for helping someone to heal trauma, it is not appropriate for everyone. How helpful it is depends on the individual, their level of trauma, and what stage of the healing process they are in. Some people may find writing about a trauma re-traumatizing. Recent studies also suggest that individuals who tend to be emotionally stoic find writing about trauma less helpful in promoting healing, whereas people who are more comfortable being emotionally open are more likely to benefit.

If you do choose to write about a trauma in your life, it's important to pay attention to how writing about the experience is affecting you. If you are feeling overwhelmed or otherwise upset, take a break for as long as you need. Do not to force yourself to write.

What's more, if you are suffering from serious trauma symptoms, it's important that you seek help from a qualified professional, such as a therapist, counselor or psychiatrist. While expressive writing may help you process your experience and emotions, using it without professional support and assistance may make you feel worse.

It's also important to bear in mind that a traumatic experience often functions to make us feel isolated, distrusting, and disconnected from other people. As a result, you might feel afraid to reach out for help. But an essential part of the healing process is breaking your isolation and creating positive social connections. For this reason, while writing can be a critical part of your healing, if you are doing it alone without any other support it could worsen your feelings of disconnection. Sharing your feelings with people you can trust—friends, family or trained professionals—usually aids recovery.

Writing Exercises

Based on research and my own experience of leading expressive writing groups for trauma survivors, the following exercises help you explore any traumatic experiences in your life, to process and understand them, and to aid your recovery and healing. As you write, don't censor yourself. However, if, at any point, your writing feels too painful or the emotions that it brings up feel overwhelming, put the writing on hold. You can always come back to it when you feel ready.

Exercise One: Write to Heal

The following exercise is adapted from exercises used in studies that have demonstrated the positive impact of expressive writing on trauma and health.

Over four consecutive days, write in a notebook about an experience that was very difficult, upsetting or challenging for you. It can be the same experience each time you write, or you can write about a different experience on different days. When you write, express your deepest thoughts and feelings. Write for about 20 minutes each time.

Because this exercise may be challenging, be gentle with yourself and if you feel overwhelmed while writing, it is okay to take a break. However, try not to get out of your writing flow and remember that sometimes we resist what is painful and preventing us from moving forward.

When you have completed the four days of writing, think about the following questions:

- What was the most challenging aspect of writing?
- Did the process of writing help to shift any feelings or make you feel differently about anything?
- Do you see your trauma differently after writing?
- Despite any lingering emotions, can you identify any healing that may have occurred?

If you want, feel free to write your answers to the questions above.

Exercise Two: Write to Heal and Reflect

This exercise is similar to Exercise One. You may choose to do it instead of Exercise One, or you can do both exercises if you wish. The exercise should be done over four consecutive days, 20 minutes each day.

Day One: Identify a traumatic or deeply upsetting experience in your life that you want to write about. Write about the experience for 20 minutes.

Day Two: Continue to write about the experience. Make sure to allow yourself to identify and explore the emotions that you felt at the time. Write for 20 minutes.

Day Three. Continue to write about the experience. This time, focus on how the experience has affected your life since it occurred. How did it change you? How did it impact the choices you've made since or the direction of your life? Write for 20 minutes.

Day Four: Having written about the experience for the last three days, reflect upon what you have learned. Write about any insights or revelations. Write about what you've learned and how it changes your view of events or yourself. Write for 20 minutes.

Exercise Three: Gain New Insights

Trauma is, by its nature, an immersive experience. In its aftermath we often feel helpless, blame ourselves, and feel shame for somehow not protecting ourselves. As a result, it's often difficult for us to step back and see the experience objectively, or to have the compassion for ourselves that we deserve.

This exercise helps you have a more objective view of what happened and, as a result, lessen the feelings of self-blame, shame or guilt that you might have. It is designed to be done over three days.

Day One: Think about a traumatic or upsetting experience. Write about it, recalling what happened, your thoughts and feelings. Write for 20 minutes.

Day Two: Go back to the time and place of the experience you wrote about yesterday. See the scene in your mind's eye. Now take a few steps back. Move away from the situation to a point where you can now watch the event unfold from a distance and see yourself in the event. As you continue to watch the situation unfold to your distant self, try to understand their feelings. Why did they have those feelings? Why did they respond in the ways that they did? If it helps, you might choose to write about yourself in third person. Write for 20 minutes.

Day Three: Reread what you wrote on day one and two. Now write about what you've learned about yourself and your experience. Write for 20 minutes.

Exercise Four: Create Self-Compassion

This exercise helps you obtain some perspective on a traumatic experience and support your healing.

Write a letter to your earlier self that experienced a trauma. Write from the perspective or yourself today. Write about what you'd say to comfort that person. What advice would you give? What would you say to that self so they no longer blame themselves for what happened? You might begin your writing with, "Dear younger self," or, "Dear 11-year-old me." Write for as long as you need.

Exercise Five: Write a Letter to the Person Who Hurt You

Sometimes it helps to get our feelings out about the person who hurt, abused or assaulted us. These feelings may be complicated, particularly if the person who hurt us was someone close to us (e.g. a parent or family member). Sometimes we may feel afraid at the extent of our rage or pain. Getting these emotions down on paper can feel cleansing and healing.

In this exercise, write a letter to the person who hurt you. In most cases, people don't plan to send these letters. Instead, this letter provides a place where you can put down all your feelings towards this person. As you write, try to avoid judging yourself for having these feelings. Just get them out. Write for as long as you need to.

If more than one person hurt you in the past, you may want to repeat this exercise so you can write to each specific person.

Sometimes, after completing this exercise, people find it useful to burn or otherwise destroy the letter. It provides a powerful symbol of letting go and can help you move on with your life.

Exercise Six: Reflecting on Trauma's Impact

A traumatic experience always changes us—sometimes in small ways, sometimes in ways that are much larger. This exercise helps you reflect on the ways that your experience of trauma impacted you. You can do it over three days, or in a single sitting. Total time is about an hour.

Step One: Write about all the ways that the trauma you experienced has influenced your life. Think about family, relationships, career, living situation, etc. Write for 20 minutes.

Step Two: In what ways are you more vulnerable as a result of this trauma? In what ways are you stronger? Write for 20 minutes.

Step Three: What have you learned by going through this trauma that now affects the way you make decisions and how you live your life? What are its negative impacts? What are its positive impacts? Write for 20 minutes.

Exercise Seven: Create a Success Journal

If you've been victimized, it may be particularly difficult to connect with the aspects of yourself that are capable and powerful. This is a very normal and understandable response to trauma. An essential part of healing is reclaiming our sense of agency and our belief in ourselves as capable of success.

To help you reconnect with that side of yourself, keep a success journal. Use a notebook or create a file on your computer, whichever works best for you. At the end of each day, write for at least five minutes about a success you experienced that day. It might be something small—for example, if you've been feeling so upset you haven't laughed and today you made a joke or experienced a moment of joy, this is a success. It could be an accomplishment at work, or doing something that you were previously fearful of, or following through with your exercise or healthy eating plan.

When you write about the success, focus on the positive feelings that come from this accomplishment. Do not let yourself veer into negative self-talk or berating yourself for not doing something more. If you find yourself doing this, redirect your writing, or simply stop until you come back the next day to write about another success.

Over time, keeping your success journal will help you notice your own assets, skills and capability. It helps build your confidence and agency—an essential part of your recovery.

Journaling: Prompts to Promote Healing

If you are healing from an experience of trauma, a journal can be a powerful and transformative companion on that journey. The following prompts help you explore and articulate your emotions, gain insight, increase your self-compassion, and support your overall healing.

You are not required to write every day, although you may find this helpful, and you do not have to do these prompts in any particular order. They are designed to help you give voice to your feelings and experience. I recommend that you take between 10 to 20 minutes on each prompt, but this is only a guideline and you can write for as much time as you want.

Bear in mind that these may bring up difficult feelings. It's fine to take a break if you are feeling overwhelmed. Do not force yourself to write. And, if you need to, make sure that you reach out to friends, family and/or professionals who can offer you support.

- These are the secrets I never told….
- When I think of my childhood self, I feel….
- The tales my body can tell.
- There was nothing I could do but…
- These are the things I would tell my (pick an age, e.g. 10-year-old) self.

- I am angry because….
- These are the things that I lost.
- This is what makes me stronger.
- I did not deserve it because….
- You let me down because….
- I should have been protected by…
- The stories I cannot share with anyone.
- The moment of fear.
- I kept quiet because….
- I told the truth because….
- I am so angry at (name of person) because….
- I am disappointed in (name of person) because….
- All the ways that I am strong.
- I am a survivor because….
- Make a list of all your strengths, skills and talents.
- Make a list of your positive qualities.
- Write about a time when you fought for yourself.
- Write about how your trauma changed you.
- I would do things differently now because….
- The things you do not know about me….
- I love myself because.
- Write about all the things you love about your body.
- The world let me down when….
- My family let me down when….
- No one should have to….
- Write about what healing means to you.
- Write about the person you want to become.
- Write a letter to the part of yourself that remains afraid or ashamed or self-blaming. Explain to that self how she or he is strong, and doesn't deserve to feel ashamed or to blame her/himself.
- Why I'm going to tell my secrets.
- Breaking free of pain.
- Becoming my true self.
- No longer living a lie.
- When fear was my friend.
- These are the things I love.
- These are the things that give me pleasure.
- Write about a time when you spoke up.

CHAPTER SIX
WRITE THROUGH GRIEF AND LOSS

"Give sorrow words. The grief that does not speak whispers the o'er-fraught heart and bids it break."

William Shakespeare, *Macbeth*

Grief is a fundamental life experience and one that all of us will almost inevitably have at some time. It is also an experience that is very individual and often overwhelming and difficult to explain. We generally think of grief arising from the death of a family member, friend, or animal companion, but it can also be triggered by the loss of a job, home, health, or a dramatic change in life circumstances that results in significant loss. In all these situations, we have to adapt to a new life and come to terms with our loss.

For some, grief may be complicated by having had a difficult or challenging relationship with the person we have lost—for example, a parent who was emotionally absent or abusive. In other cases, sadness may be accompanied by contradictory feelings—for example, it's normal for a person who was a full-time caregiver for a terminally ill person to have some feelings of relief after the death of their loved one.

Studies have shown that expressive writing can help people move through grief and come to terms with loss. It offers us a way to articulate and understand our emotions and for us to find meaning in the experience.

Writing doesn't make our sadness go away immediately and in the short term it may sharpen our emotions and make them more intense. For this reason, it's important to do the exercises below at your own pace and in a way that feels manageable to you. If you find yourself feeling overwhelmed or are experiencing depression or other serious symptoms, it is important to reach out for help from a counselor, therapist, or through a grief support group.

A Journal to Move through Grief

You may want to keep a journal or a notebook where you write about how you feel about your loss. You can simply write about your day, your feelings and thoughts. Or you can use some more structured approaches to help you cope with grief. One suggestion from therapist Kathleen Adams is to get in the habit of writing three words that describe your feelings at the beginning and end of every journal entry. This helps you track your feelings over time and allows you to notice how you are moving through your grief.

Because grief can often feel overwhelming and impact how we are able to take care of ourselves, it can also be a good idea to use your journal to actively support your well-being. To do this, Adams suggests that before you go to bed you think of something you'd like to experience the next day—a small pleasure, an experience such as a walk or a productive meeting at work. Write this experience in your journal and also write a few notes on what you can do to arrange your day to increase the likelihood that your choice will manifest. The following evening, write for five minutes about what happened and what you learned.

While it's perfectly fine to use your journal to write whatever comes into your mind, be aware that if you use your journal only to ruminate on depressive thoughts or negative feelings about yourself, this can undermine your mental and physical health. Try to notice if you are turning your natural feelings of sadness into negative self-talk. If this is the case, it may be a good time to reach out to friends, family, or a professional for support.

The prompts below help you focus your writing and move through the emotions that come with loss. You can write for as long as you want, but if it makes it easier to have a specific time to stop, decide on something that works for you.

You may choose to do the exercises in order, or just those that appeal to you. And, because it can take time for us to metabolize our feelings of grief, you may find that you want to do all or some of the exercises more than once. In all cases, write freely and without judgement and don't worry about spelling or grammar—simply focus on getting your thoughts and feelings onto the page.

- Write a description of the person (or animal companion, place, life situation) you have lost.

- Write an obituary for the person (or animal companion, place, life situation) you have lost.

- Write about the first time you met the person you have lost.

- Write a story about an important occasion spent with the person you have lost.

- Write about a happy memory involving the person (or animal companion, place, life situation) you have lost.

- Write a letter to the person you have lost. Tell them all the things you wish you had told them when you could.

- If you had a difficult or challenging relationship with the person you lost, it's very normal to have negative or conflicted feelings towards them. Write about those feelings.

- Think about all the ways the person you have lost (or animal companion, place, life situation) affected your life and changed you in positive ways. Write about these things. You can write it in the form of a letter if that feels right to you.

- Write about all the things you are grateful for that resulted from knowing the person (or animal companion, place, life situation) you lost.

- Think about your grief. Imagine it as a kind of weather (e.g. a snowstorm, a rainy day, thick fog). Describe that weather in detail.

- Write about something you experienced in your day that reminded you of the person you have lost (or animal companion, place, life situation).

- Write about guilt and feeling guilty.

- Write about despair.

- Write about the things that give you comfort or make you feel joy.

- Write the story of your relationship with the person you have lost. Begin your story with, "Once upon a Time…."

- Make a list of everything you miss about the person you have lost.

- Think about the person (or animal companion) you have lost and what was important to them. Write about one thing you'd like to do to honor them and who they were. This could be, for example, a private goodbye ritual, volunteering at an organization they supported, or taking a trip to a place you visited together. Or it could be something else entirely. Write about what makes most sense for you.

Accepting and Honoring our Feelings of Loss

Sometimes we get subtle or not-so-subtle messages from others that we are "too sad" or too affected by our loss. This is, in part, because many people are uncomfortable when dealing with grief, death and loss. Mainstream western society does a very poor job of dealing with death and tends to minimize the emotional toll that grief can take on an individual. Many employers think they are being generous when they offer three days' bereavement leave!

In other cases, many of those around us may not recognize the significance of our loss. Despite recent advances in LGBT rights, same-sex relationships are still seen by many as less significant or meaningful than heterosexual partnerships. For some, the loss of an animal companion can be devastating, but non-pet lovers may have difficulty understanding the depth of their grief. And if you have been affected by the loss of a job, your home, or something else, others may not realize the extent of its impact on you. So it's no surprise that we may engage in self-talk telling us to "just get over it" or "move on."

The fact is that the grief process takes time and it is different for everyone. It cannot be hurried or expedited. In fact, if we try to do this, we will likely end up suppressing our feelings. Those suppressed feelings can end up harming our health.

The following exercise helps foster self-compassion and honor our feelings of loss. Write freely and without censoring yourself. You can do all the steps in one sitting or you can do them over three days. Total time is about an hour.

Step One: Think about all the things that have changed in your life as a result of your loss. Write about your feelings about these changes. Write for 20 minutes.

Step Two: Imagine that a kind and supportive friend just read over what you wrote in step one. Imagine what words of comfort, support and encouragement that they might offer you. Write down what they say. Write for 20 minutes.

Step Three: Read over slowly what you wrote in step two and let the words really sink in. Let yourself feel the support, compassion and acceptance that the friend offered you. Now write about what you can do to offer yourself this kind of support yourself. Write for 10 to 20 minutes.

Keep what you wrote in steps two and three. You can review it whenever you are feeling critical of yourself and how you are coping.

CHAPTER SEVEN
WRITE TO SUPPORT OPTIMISM AND A POSITIVE OUTLOOK

"Through writing, we revisit our past and review and revise it. What we thought happened, what we believed happened to us, shifts and changes as we discover deeper and more complex truths. It isn't that we use our writing to deny what we've experienced. Rather, we use it to shift our perspective."

Louise DeSalvo, *Writing as a Way of Healing.*

For all humans, there are certain basic needs we must address (such as food, shelter, sleep, and safety) that allow us to live satisfying lives. But, despite what we're told every day in advertisements, on the internet and in glossy magazines, above a certain income threshold, earning more money and having more material goods makes little difference in how happy we feel.

The field of positive psychology has examined what ingredients help people create happy and fulfilled lives. One of the key things they identified was a positive outlook. This doesn't mean that you ignore life's troubles or the larger social issues that give you concern. It means being more optimistic and looking for the good in things rather than being a pessimist or a cynic and concentrating on the bad. Cultivating a positive outlook means that you'll have a better experience of yourself. You'll also likely find that other people want to spend more time with you. This helps build social connection—another key element strongly associated with happiness and fulfillment.

Journaling for Optimism

Studies have shown that it's possible to cultivate a positive outlook through expressive writing. One of the things that's proven particularly successful is keeping a gratitude journal (see Chapter Three). A gratitude journal allows you to focus on what's good in your life and what you appreciate. Over time, it can help you develop a more positive outlook overall. Sometimes, people decide to keep a gratitude journal on an indefinite basis, but you can also decide on a specific amount of time—a month or three months, for example—to cultivate this practice.

One option for a gratitude journal is to focus on writing about things in the natural world that you are grateful for. Connecting to nature has been shown to have an extremely positive effect on outlook, and noticing aspects of nature in your daily life and writing about them can boost your mental health. You might, for example, choose to write about the beauty of storm clouds or a sunset, the birds chirping outside your window, the way the sunlight reflects on a puddle, or the smell of the flowers blooming in a neighbor's yard. This practice also helps us be present in the moment (you might find yourself literally stopping to smell the roses) and develop a more mindful approach to life, which has also been shown to increase positive outlook and overall health.

Another possibility is to create a "humor journal," that is, a daily writing practice in which you write one or more funny things that you experienced during your day. You might write about something you were directly involved in or something you observed. This could be an incident that made you laugh at the time or something that, upon reflection, seems humorous. This practice can be particularly helpful if you have a habit of being very self-critical or taking yourself and life a little too seriously. Humor helps us rebound from challenges in part because we're less likely to see them as disasters and instead regard them as just the funny ups and downs of life.

In addition to journaling to support optimism, there are other writing techniques that can help you create more happiness in your life. The exercises below help support this goal. As is the case with the other exercises in this book, write freely without judging or censoring yourself, don't worry about spelling or grammar, just focus on getting the words on the page.

Exercise: Cultivate an Optimistic Outlook

Think about a current problem or challenge that is playing on your mind. This could be an upcoming job interview, an approaching vacation with your difficult in-laws, a stressful project at work, or a recent health exam that gave you cause for concern. You can do this exercise in a single sitting or over three days. Total time is 30 to 60 minutes.

Step One: Once you have this problem in mind, imagine the most positive outcome possible for this event. For example, you get the job, or the vacation with the in-laws ends up being fun. In as much detail as possible, write about that positive outcome and what happens as a result. Write for 10 to 20 minutes.

Step Two: With the same problem in mind, imagine that there is a negative outcome. You don't get the job, the vacation doesn't go so well. Now, think about what the "silver lining" of such an outcome might be. Write about that silver lining. Write for about 10 to 20 minutes.

Step Three: Review what you wrote in steps one and two. Now write about what you learned and how your attitude towards this problem has changed. Write for 10 to 20 minutes.

You can repeat this exercise for any problem that is bothering you. It will likely help you change how you perceive the problem. What's more, over time, if you repeat this exercise, it will help you start to reframe what you once saw as "problems" into "opportunities" to grow and change.

Exercise: Letting Go of Negative Emotions

It's natural to feel anger or sadness or other difficult emotions. It's also appropriate to feel angry when someone hurts us, or sad if we experience a loss. But sometimes we hold on to these emotions for too long. They can get in the way of enjoying our everyday lives and potentially interfere with our success in relationships or career.

This exercise helps you let go of these emotions and move on. Please note that this will likely not happen immediately, but you may find your feelings shifting over time. It's possible to do this exercise more than once if you need to explore an experience or emotion that has been really holding you back. You can do this exercise in a single sitting or over three days. Total time is 30 to 60 minutes.

Step One: Think about what negative emotion you may be holding on to. Perhaps it's anger at a past hurt or pain and sadness at a loss. Think about the experience that prompted that emotion. Write about that experience for 10 to 20 minutes.

Step Two: Think about the experience you wrote about in step one. But this time, think about the positive things you may have gleaned from that experience. Perhaps it made you stronger or wiser. Perhaps it motivated you to change your behaviors or attitudes in a positive way. Write about those positive things that came out of the experience. Write for 10 to 20 minutes.

Step Three: Review what you wrote in step one and two. Now think about what you think you need to do to let go of the negative emotions that resulted from that experience. Write about what you will do to let go of those feelings. Write for 10 to 20 minutes.

Exercise: Creating Self-Compassion

Self-compassion means that you treat yourself with care and concern when confronted with your own mistakes, failures and shortcomings. Having compassion for ourselves helps us feel better because we're less likely to be tortured by a negative inner voice.

This exercise helps you nurture self-compassion. You can do it in a single sitting or over three days. Total time is 30 to 60 minutes.

Step One: Start by thinking of an aspect of yourself that you dislike and criticize. It could be something about your appearance, a habit, your career, your relationships, or your health. Write in detail about how this perceived inadequacy makes you feel. Write the thoughts, images, emotions, or stories that come up when you think about it. Write for 10 to 20 minutes.

Step Two: Imagine a friend who is unconditionally loving, accepting, and supportive. This friend sees your strengths and opportunities for growth, including the negative aspects about you. The friend accepts and forgives you, embracing you kindly just as you are. Write a letter to yourself from the perspective of this kind friend. Write what this friend says to support or encourage you. Write what steps they suggest you take to change. Write for 10 to 20 minutes.

Step Three: Put what you wrote in step two aside for at least 20 minutes. When you return to it, read it over slowly and let the words really sink in. Let yourself feel the support, compassion and acceptance that the friend offered you. Now write about what you can do to offer yourself this kind of support. Write for 10 to 20 minutes.

Keep what you wrote in step two and three. You can review it whenever you are feeling down about this aspect and remember that accepting yourself is the first step to change.

Exercise: Imagine Your Best Possible Self

This exercise has been shown to improve people's mood, optimism and well-being. It is also an exercise you can repeat and is particularly helpful when you are feeling negatively about your life or yourself and want to shift those feelings. You can do it in a single sitting or over two days. Total time is 20 to 40 minutes.

Step One: Think about your best possible future self. Picture that you have performed to the best of your abilities and you had achieved the things you wanted to in life. Describe this person in detail. Write for 10 to 20 minutes.

Step Two: After completing step one, reflect on your feelings and answer the following questions: How did it motivate or inspire you? What did it make you want to change now? Write for 10 to 20 minutes.

Elaine Beale

CHAPTER EIGHT
WRITE TO CREATE POSITIVE RELATIONSHIPS AT HOME AND WORK

"Expression empowers us to transform our feelings; it permits us to connect our stories with the stories of others, to bridge the gulf of our essential isolation from one another."

Gabriele Rico, *Pain and Possibility: Writing Your Way Through Personal Crisis.*

Numerous studies show that having poor social connections is associated with a higher mortality risk. In fact, recent research indicates that loneliness might be a more significant health factor than obesity, smoking, exercise, or nutrition. Thus, the number and quality of our relationships is a key wellness issue that we would do well to pay attention to.

Expressive writing has been shown to help support stability in the relationships of married couples. It has also been shown to have a healing effect for couples struggling with infidelity or emotional trauma. It can improve our communication with romantic partners, spouses, as well as other important people in our lives. It is thought that this comes, at least in part, from the fact that by writing down our thoughts and feelings we can see our role in relationships more clearly and can also more easily empathize with another's point-of-view.

Thus, writing can not only improve our most intimate relationships, but it can also help us to have more harmonious relationships with family members, work colleagues, and friends. And having these positive relationships can improve our happiness and satisfaction. Additionally, less conflict and more positive social attachments can create lasting improvements in our physical health.

Keeping a journal on an ongoing basis can be very helpful in maintaining positive relationships. In some instances, simply getting our negative feelings onto the page means we are less likely to blow up at others. A journal can also help us keep track of our emotions in our relationships. This can be a great tool in helping us identify when a relationship we're involved in is toxic or abusive. It can also help us identify patterns in our own behavior that result in conflict or cause us to get involved in unhealthy dynamics with other people in our lives.

The following exercises help you resolve conflicts more easily, develop greater empathy, and generally improve your relationships with significant others, family, friends and co-workers.

Exercise: Resolve Conflicts

If you are experiencing a conflict or feeling frustrated or angry with someone in your life, this exercise can help you gain some perspective and potentially gain insight into what actions you might take to resolve the conflict. It's best if you do this exercise over four consecutive days.

Day One: Think about the conflict or the situation that is causing you to feel angry or frustrated. Write about it, focusing on how you feel rather than on the details of what happened. Write for 10 to 20 minutes.

Days Two through Four: Repeat this exercise three more times, focusing on the same conflict or situation. Continue to focus on your feelings. Each time, write for 10 to 20 minutes.

Day Five: Once you have written about the conflict four times, review what you have written. Now take some time to write about any insights or revelations you may have had about the situation. Write for about 20 minutes.

Exercise: See Another's Point of View

When you are not seeing eye to eye with a partner, friend or co-worker, it can be easy to feel aggrieved and find it difficult to let go of anger. This exercise helps you look at a situation or conflict from the point of view of the other person involved. It may help you develop more understanding of the overall situation and make it easier to let go of resentment or anger. You can do this exercise in a single sitting or over three days. Total time is 30 to 60 minutes.

Step One: Think about the conflict that is bothering you. Write about it as you see it. Write about how you feel and go as deeply into your emotions as you can. Write for 10 to 20 minutes.

Step Two: This time when you think of the conflict, instead of looking at it from your perspective, think about it from the other person's point of view. Write about what you think they might be feeling and why. Stay in that point of view as you write for 10 to 20 minutes.

Step Three: Reread what you wrote in steps one and two. Reflect on any insights or revelations that you may have had about the conflict or situation. Write about these insights and how they might change how you approach the conflict going forward. Write for 10 to 20 minutes.

Exercise: Resolving Feelings about Relationships

Sometimes we carry around negative emotions about people in our past or about people we interact with in our present lives. When we carry around these unresolved feelings, it can sour our current relationships and also make life more difficult for ourselves. This exercise helps you understand and let go of those feelings.

Step One: Make a list of everyone you're angry with and why.

Step Two: Identify the person that you are most angry with. Write a letter to that person (this is not to be given to or read to that person, it is a tool to help you process your anger). Be completely candid in your letter, describing what your feelings are and what you need to say. The letter is for your eyes only and should be written with complete honesty. Take as long as you need to write the letter.

Sometimes, people who do this exercise find it useful to burn, bury or otherwise destroy their letter. This can be helpful in allowing you to let go of your anger.

Once you have completed your letter to the person you are most angry with, you may want to pick a second person on the list and go through the same process with them.

You can choose to do this same exercise for people you feel that you need to forgive, or for people whom you have wronged and from whom you need to ask forgiveness. There may also be people in your life with whom you have unresolved emotional business and you can follow the same process for them, too.

CHAPTER NINE
WRITE FOR SELF-DEVELOPMENT AND INSIGHT

"Expressive and explorative writing is really a process of deep listening, attending to some of the many aspects of the self habitually blanketed during waking lives."

Gillian Bolton, *Write Yourself: Creative Writing and Personal Development*

In today's busy world, we spend much of our time being barraged with sensory and informational input. Silence, solitude and reflection are not highly valued in contemporary society. As a result, most of us rarely take the time to really examine our thoughts and emotions.

One of the amazing things about expressive writing is that it provides a window into your deepest self. By writing without censoring yourself, you connect with the wisdom and insight provided by your unconscious mind. This allows you to become acquainted with the self that lies below the surface. You learn about your true desires, discover valuable revelations, and, as a result, can make wiser and more conscious choices about your life priorities and goals.

The following exercises allow you to gain deeper insight into yourself, your life and what's important to you. You can do all of them or some of them, but it is likely that the more of the exercises you do, the more you will connect to your intuitive, creative self and the more you will learn.

As with all the other exercises in this book, you should write as freely as possible and try not to censor yourself.

Exercise One: Your Life Story
Write the story of your life. You can start with your birth, or conception, or at a later stage of your life. Write for as long as you want.

Exercise Two: Your Life Story in Third Person
Write the story of your life. This time, write it in third person (he/she) rather than first person. Start at whatever stage of your life you want to. Write for as long as you want.

Exercise Three: Dig Deeper
The following prompts are springboards for you to dive in and get to know yourself more deeply. Pick whichever prompts appeal to you and write for as long as you want. Remember, there's no right way to do this exercise, just write whatever comes into your head. Also, many of these prompts can be repeated several times since they are likely to evoke different feelings and memories each time you write.

- I believe….
- I always thought that….
- I never thought that….
- I remember….
- I don't remember….
- I was always told….
- I believe….
- I don't believe….
- I feel…
- I want….
- I wish….
- I can….
- If I could do it over again, I would….
- I most regret….
- I don't regret….
- I won't forget…
- I wish I could forget….
- More than anything, I value….
- If I ruled the world….
- I love….
- I hate….
- I care about….
- I don't care about….

Exercise Four: Life Events
Take a few minutes to make a list of the major events in your life. Once you

have made a list of those events, choose one. Write about it for 10 to 20 minutes.

If you wish, you can choose several of the events on your list and write about them. Write about each of them for 10 to 20 minutes.

When you are done writing about all the events you want to write about, read over what you have written. Take as long as you want to write about how you feel.

Exercise Five: The People in Your Life

Take a few minutes to make a list of the most important people in your life. Once you have made a list of those people, choose one. Write about that person for 10 to 20 minutes.

If you wish, you can choose several of the people on your list and write about them. Write about each of them for 10 to 20 minutes.

When you are done writing about all the people you want to write about, read over what you have written. Take as long as you want to write about how you feel.

Exercise Six: The Places in Your Life

Take a few minutes to make a list of the most important places in your life. Once you have made a list of those places, choose one. Write about them for 10 to 20 minutes.

If you wish, you can choose several of the places on your list and write about them. Write about each of them for 10 to 20 minutes.

When you are done writing about all the places you want to write about, read over what you have written. Take as long as you want to write about how you feel.

Exercise Seven: The Objects in Your Life

Take a few minutes to make a list of the most important things in your life. (These could include childhood toys, a piece of jewelry, a car, your bike, a stone you found on the beach, or whatever objects have significance for you. If you have a difficult time deciding, imagine that your home is on fire and, in addition to important papers and practical items, you can only take four additional objects. What would these be?) Once you have made a list of those objects, choose one. Write about it for 10 to 20 minutes.

If you wish, you can choose several of the items on your list and write about them. Write about each of them for 10 to 20 minutes.

When you are done writing about all the things you want to write about, read over what you have written. Take as long as you want to write about how you feel.

Exercise Eight: Lessons from Childhood

The following prompts get you to write about your childhood. After writing in response to several prompts, you may find that themes arise, or that you make connections between events in the past and those that are happening now. You may gain insights about events or people in your childhood that influenced you. Or you may find yourself writing memories that you had thought you had forgotten but that have great resonance for you. Choose from any of the prompts that appeal to you. Write for 10 to 20 minutes each time.

- Your bedroom
- The house you grew up in
- Learning to tie your shoes
- Favorite foods
- First day of school
- Learning to read
- Favorite games
- Best friends
- Bullies
- Family dinners
- Playing games
- Summer evenings
- Winter nights
- Holidays
- A teacher
- On the way to school
- Favorite candy
- Imaginary friends
- Puberty
- First kiss
- Birthdays
- My mother
- My father
- The things I was told
- The things I learned

Exercise Nine: Turning Points

It is often possible to identify distinct turning points or moments of significant transformation in our lives. Sometimes these changes come at times when we might most expect them: graduation from school, a marriage, the birth of a child, the death of a parent. But sometimes these turning points come unexpectedly and it is only when looking back that we can identify them.

This exercise helps you identify key turning points in your life and their significance. You can do this exercise in a single sitting or over the course of two days. Total time is up to an hour.

Step One: Think about an event or series of events in your life that changed everything. Write about what happened. Write for up to 30 minutes.

Step Two: Read what you wrote in step one. Think about how that turning point affected you and its impact on your life and who you are now. Write about it for up to 30 minutes.

Elaine Beale

CHAPTER TEN
CREATE A WELLNESS WRITING GROUP

"There is no greater agony than bearing an untold story within you."
Maya Angelou

It isn't necessary to be in a group to gain benefit from any of the exercises in this book, but writing with a group of others can be a powerful and useful experience. It can:

- Keep you writing regularly.
- Provide structure and accountability to support your writing practice and keep you focused on your health, self-care and/or healing.
- Connect you to people who have similar experiences, priorities or interests as you.
- Provide emotional support when you're writing about challenging issues such as illness, grief or trauma.
- Provide a place where you can share your writing if you want to.
- Writing with others can sometimes help people go deeper and explore emotions or experiences that they may not be comfortable exploring alone.

In the groups that I've led, I've witnessed participants go through startling transformations as they write, share what they've written, and receive feedback, support, and affirmation from other members of the group.

Since groups that use expressive writing as a tool for health and healing are not offered in many communities, if you want to participate in this kind of group, you will likely have to set up your own. In some cases, you may have a group of friends who want to create a wellness writing group with you. But in many cases, particularly if you want to write about a specific theme (such as living with chronic illness or dealing with grief), you may need to reach out into your community to create a group. If you've never set up a group before, this can feel a little intimidating. For this reason, I've devoted this chapter to providing guidelines you can use to set up and run a wellness writing group.

Identify Your Target Group

When you're putting together your group, you should think first about who you'd like to be in it and the purpose of the group. When identifying who you're targeting, be as specific as you need. For example, if you have been recently diagnosed with fibromyalgia you may want to bring together a group of people living with that disease. It might be, however, that you want to target a wider group—say, people living with chronic illness. Things to bear in mind as you decide upon your target group include:

- The size of your community (if you live in a small community, you may need to make your target audience wider to get enough group members);
- How gender, age, race, or other demographics might impact the group and whether you want to target a specific demographic. You may, for example, feel that you'd like to create a group that targets women with cancer because of the specific issues and concerns women may experience.

It's also important to define your group's purpose so, when you are recruiting potential members, you can find people who share your interests or goals. For example, this could be a group for women recently diagnosed with cancer who want to use expressive writing to improve their quality of life. Or it might be a group for survivors of sexual trauma who want to use writing to support their healing. Or it could be a group for caregivers who want to use writing to help them cope with isolation and stress.

Remember, the more clearly you can define your group's purpose and the people you want to recruit, the more likely you are to reach them.

Recruiting Your Group

Once you've decided upon your target population and purpose of your writing group, you need to recruit members. You might use Facebook, Twitter, or Instagram to get the word out. You can also list your group on sites like Craigslist or Nextdoor. You can create flyers or posters advertising the group in your community and post them in the places where your target group is likely to go. For example, if you're forming a group for people living with chronic illness, you might want to post flyers at a hospital or clinic. You can also reach out to groups or individuals who interact with your target group—for example, you might contact doctors or counselors in your community so they can refer patients or clients who might be interested. You can also post flyers or leave postcards at grocery stores, fitness centers, senior centers, yoga studios, or local colleges. The wider your reach, the more likely you are to find people interested in your group.

In your publicity, make sure to let people know the following information:

- Who you are targeting and the purpose of your group.
- Contact information.
- Place and time of meeting.
- Any other information that's relevant such as accessibility information, any costs involved.

Where, When, and How Long to Meet

Where and when you choose to meet is up to you. But bear in mind the following:

- The group will need to meet in a quiet space where you won't be disturbed.
- Try to find a public space for your meetings. There are often free meeting rooms at the public library or in a local school or college. Sometimes churches or community centers provide free or low-cost rooms.
- If you can't locate a community space and you find you need to meet in a private home, you may want to have an initial get-to-know-you meeting in a public space like a café where you can meet people, discuss ground rules and other aspects of the group.
- If you do meet in a private home, you may want to consider rotating the location of the meeting so one person doesn't have to bear the burden of hosting and clean-up.
- The time of day and the week you meet will affect who is likely to be able attend—for example, evenings may not be a great time for older people while weekdays are hard for people who work.

- How often you meet depends on what makes sense for participants. Generally, the groups I lead meet weekly, but you may find that every other week or once a month work better for your group. Be aware, however, that the less frequent the meetings, the longer time it takes to build a sense of trust and ease within the group.
- I've found that the optimal length of time for a meeting is between two and two-and-a-half hours.
- It's usually a good idea to have the group meet a specific number of times. I'd recommend six times as the minimum and 12 times as the maximum. If, upon completing your planned number of meetings, the group decides it wants to continue, you can always add another round of meetings.
- While it is possible to run an expressive writing group as a drop-in group (i.e. people drop in when they want, rather than make a commitment to attend every meeting), this will make it challenging to create the kind of safety and trust that's required for people to feel at ease enough to write emotionally difficult material and to share that material with the group. For this reason, I strongly suggest you create a closed group that members commit to attend for a specific number of meetings.

Facilitation

It's important to have someone who acts as the group facilitator. If you are meeting with a group of peers (i.e. you don't have a professional in the facilitator role), I encourage you to rotate this role from week to week. Generally, the responsibility of this person is to:

- Plan what exercises and prompts you will use for the meeting.
- Introduce each exercise and provide clear instructions, including how much time is allotted.
- Time each exercise (you may want to use a timer, such as the one on your cellphone) and let participants know when time is up.
- Invite participants to share their work after each exercise.
- Ensure that the group follows the guidelines to ensure that the group remains supportive and safe.
- Since some participants are usually more at ease sharing what they've written, the facilitator can also play an important role in making sure that everyone has an opportunity to read aloud. The facilitator also makes sure that the group finishes on time and that the group appoints a facilitator for the following meeting.

- The facilitator writes in response to the exercises and prompts, just like everyone else.

Ground Rules

When creating a wellness writing group, it's critically important that you observe a set of ground rules that establish the group as a supportive and safe space. This allows participants to write freely and without censoring themselves, and to explore the deep and potentially difficult emotions and experiences that will likely arise as they write. The ground rules I suggest you adopt are:

- All writing and experiences shared in the group are kept confidential.
- There is no "correct" response to any of the prompts or exercises. Participants can write whatever they wish or whatever comes up for them.
- It is always optional to share your writing. This means that while participants might encourage each other to read aloud what they've written, it is fine if someone says they want to pass. No justifications or excuses are required.
- When someone does read aloud what they have written, responses from the group should be supportive, non-judgmental, and validating.
- Often, what is shared in the group is very personal, vulnerable and revealing. For this reason, it's important that all interactions are grounded in respect, caring and compassion.
- If you do read aloud, try not to preface it with a disclaimer or a negative comment such as, "This is really badly written," or, "What I wrote is so negative," or, "I don't like this, but I suppose I'll read it." We reinforce our inner critic and self-judgment by speaking it aloud. Instead, of saying these things about yourself and your writing, try to take a breath, let go of that negative self-talk, and simply read.

It's important to establish these ground rules from the first meeting, and you may find it helpful to revisit them at the beginning of each meeting. It helps set the tone of the meeting and reinforces the idea of the group as a safe and supportive space.

Group Activities

I suggest that you use this book to find the exercises to use in your group. Depending on your group's target audience and purpose, different chapters will be relevant to you. However, most of the exercises in Chapter Three will be useful to any group, regardless of audience and purpose. You may also find that exercises in chapters not directly relating to your target group might be relevant to you. For example, if your group is for people with chronic illness, the exercises in Chapter Four will be most relevant to you, but there are also useful exercises in the Chapters Three, Seven, Eight and Nine.

If you are sharing facilitation, you can have the facilitator for that week pick out two or three exercises to complete. If you have a single facilitator over the course of your planned series of meetings, then that person can undertake long-term planning of what topics and exercises to use over the course of the group.

I'd suggest that you run each group meeting in the following sequence:

1. A brief check-in in which group members go around and talk about how they have been feeling since the last meeting and any revelations or thoughts that have arisen. (Allow about 10 to 15 minutes.)
2. A quick review of group guidelines. (Allow no more than five minutes.)
3. Write using exercises from this book. After each exercise, allow time for participants to read aloud what they've written. Remember, not everyone needs to read every time and it's always okay to pass. (Allow 1.5 to 2 hours, depending on the overall length of the group.)
4. A check-out in which group members take turns to say how they're feeling and any realizations that they may have had during the group. (Allow about 10 to 15 minutes.)

Practice Self-Care and Seek Out Support
The group itself will function as a place to help you develop greater self-compassion and practice more self-care. It will also provide social support and understanding, and you may find yourself developing friendships with other participants.

It's important to remember, however, that expressive writing can bring up challenging emotions and, at least in the short term, may make you feel worse. For this reason, I strongly suggest that you make sure you are particularly kind and attentive to yourself while participating in the group. This may mean taking extra time for pleasurable activities, letting yourself relax and do nothing, and using any tools you already use to take care of yourself (for example, walks in nature, cups of hot tea, spending time in your garden, yoga, laughing with friends, sleeping late, doing a hobby you enjoy, stroking your dog or cat).

It's also important to reach out to your existing networks if you need extra support. Perhaps let your friends or family know that you are joining the group, or give yourself permission to call a friend when the group brings up difficult emotions. You may also find that you need to reach out for more professional help—from a counselor, therapist or doctor.

Over time, I am confident that you will find writing in a group a highly effective means to support your health and wellness. It will not only offer you all the profound benefits of expressive writing, but will also connect you to a group of supportive people who are willing to honestly explore their emotions, prioritize self-knowledge, and commit to their own health.

ABOUT THE AUTHOR

Elaine Beale is an award-winning writer and published novelist. She has taught creative and expressive writing in community settings and educational institutions for more than 20 years. In addition to leading writing workshops, she coaches individual writers and provides manuscript consulting and editing services. Elaine is a Certified Professional Coach and a Certified Health Coach. She trained as an educator at the University of London in the United Kingdom, and has a Master's of Fine Arts in Creative Writing from the University of British Columbia, Canada.

Write for Wellness is based on *Write Well!*, an evidence-based program Elaine created to empower people to improve their health and wellness through the use of expressive writing. Elaine presents *Write Well!* at conferences, in workplaces, and in the community. She can be contacted through her website, www.elainebeale.com.